Lost

Lost

A True Story of Navigating the
Healthcare System Against the Tide
and Into Gastroparesis

Cynthia Williams

Library of Congress Control Number: 2010905356
ISBN: Hardcover   978-1-4500-8524-3
                   Softcover   978-1-4500-8523-6
                   Ebook   978-1-4500-8525-0

This book was printed in the United States of America.

To order additional copies of this book, contact:
Xlibris Corporation
1-888-795-4274
www.Xlibris.com
Orders@Xlibris.com
79032

This book is dedicated to all those
who have not found hope in the health care
system and to those who have overcome illness
despite the health care system

I also want to thank my husband, children,
mom, dad, and my best friends Patty
and Valerie for watching over me.

Prologue

I am two years old. I am surrounded by people I do not know. They are talking fast and touching me. I do not understand what is happening. I am scared. I keep trying to find my mommy but I can hardly see anything between all the other crisply dressed people. I hear someone say "hurry, we are losing her." How could they lose me, I am right here. I catch a glimpse of my mommy. She is standing alone in the corner of the room. She is crying.

It is dark now. I am lost.

As I open my eyes, I see my mommy first. She looks so tired. I try to speak but my voice is so soft and my throat is burning. Mommy comes to me and gives me a big hug. She is crying again but this time the tears are of joy, not fear. I am in a hospital. The crib I am in is surrounded by a plastic tent. There is a soft swooshing sound of oxygen being circulated in the tent. All I want to do is go home and play.

I have asthma and I just survived cardiac arrest due to respiratory failure. This is the only time I experienced cardiac arrest but I have a lifelong journey in front of me, with asthma defining the boundaries of my abilities.

Chapter 1

As a teenager, the years were tumultuous and rebellious. I was a strong-headed independent teen who clearly did not have the maturity or life experiences to make sound decisions. I chose friends that I believed I could trust but boys, well that was a different story. My closest friend lived right down the road. Her family structure was very different from mine. She lived with her mom and her older sister. Her mom's boyfriend lived in the other half of the house but it could have been across the town for all I knew about him. They were a very open family. They talked about everything. Some conversations surprised me into silence, especially when they talked about sex. I was a naive girl trying to be worldly. I was barely treading water but acting like the captain of the ship.

Just like any other teenager, I thought my parents were overbearing and strict. I could not comprehend that they had rules to protect me. I thought they had rules just to make my life miserable. I rebelled. I dated the "bad boy" types. They did not come into the house and meet my parents before a date. They smoked, drank, and drove beat-up old cars too fast. I stayed out late, drank with them, and even tried marijuana and cocaine. At one point, either by the insistence of my mom or just as coincidence, my asthma doctor told me that smoking marijuana could kill me because of the relaxation effect and that I would not be able to struggle and overcome an asthma attack. I never smoked it again.

I attended a private school for the first two years of high school. It was an elite school, and a lot of the other kids came from really big money. There were these two brothers that I got to know as friends. One was a rowdy bad boy and the other was a stunning, well-mannered athlete. Their parents would pick them up for school break in a personal jet. Other parents were ambassadors, senators, and doctors. My parents owned the country store in the center of town. Although owning that store was a magnificent achievement and certainly something to be proud of, I did not see it that way. To me, we were the poor people and I was able to attend the school as a charity case. I had no idea how things really were. It never dawned on me that the school was expensive and my parents made the payments so I could have the advantage of an exceptional education. I wore fancy clothes as we needed to dress up to go to school. I never questioned the expense of the clothes. It was to me just the way things were. My dad drove old used cars, and I was embarrassed by that. We lived in an old colonial house on the main road in town. That was something I was proud of. Somehow I knew that the house was a prize and I was lucky to be there. I walked to school each morning. Well, more like strutted to school. I walked home each evening around five, because the school required sport participation after school. I did minimal homework because I had more important things to do, like hang out with my friends. I would skip classes or skip the whole day. My parents always found out so one would think I would learn my lesson. But I did not.

My parents took me to counseling after the first time I ran away from home. I was staying at the friend's house that was just down the road. I could not at the time possibly comprehend the fear and anguish that I caused my parents. Not only had I run away but after being with me year in and year out watching me struggle and suffer to overcome multiple asthma attacks, my mother must have been in a state of absolute terror. What if something happened and no one around me knew what to do? But I, with my infinite teenage wisdom, thought nothing of it.

When I was a child, my doctor at the time told my mother that she had two choices. She could limit my activity and essentially have me live in a bubble, so to speak, or allow me to find my own limitations through trial and error. My mother chose option two although it must have been a difficult and heart-wrenching decision. For her it meant standing back and allowing me to become ill as I tried activities and found what I could and could not tolerate. For me it was empowering. I found I could do a lot of things like swimming, soccer, softball, and even some long distance running if the weather was good and I paced myself. I grew up believing there really wasn't anything I couldn't do. I was just like all the other kids.

At the same time, I ended up in and out of the hospital with asthma attacks. They came on for many different reasons—a cold, too much activity, exposure to dogs and cats, and even the change of seasons, although all doctors at the time told my mother the weather does not trigger asthma. But like clockwork I would be in the hospital in the fall as the days were warm and the nights were cold. I would again be in the hospital every January as the weather dipped into a deep freeze. This was such a curse as my birthday is in the middle of January. But the worst year was when I was in the hospital for Christmas.

That year was particularly bad. The asthma attack I had was severe and I was in the hospital for over a week. On Christmas eve my dad came to visit me. He told me that he saw Santa in the parking lot as he was coming in. He told Santa he would be happy to give me my presents as he was headed to my room anyhow. I believed him as I was only four. He brought me pop-together blocks and I played with them in my hospital bed for hours. As far as I recall, that was the only time my dad came to the hospital alone. He always came with my mom.

My mom was always there, no matter what. There were multiple trips to the emergency room late at night, on weekends and holidays. One Christmas there was an hors d'oeuvres of mixed nuts and raisins. I tried some and found out I was allergic to nuts. I had an anaphylactic reaction and scared the whole family. I was allergic to so many things that my mother had to eliminate all foods and start with just potatoes and slowly add new foods to determine what I was allergic to. That was definitely not a fun summer. But all in all, I managed to make it to adolescence.

As a teenager, hormones, emotions, and just plain stubbornness ruled my world. I think I am the sole cause of my mother's gray hair. I know I was unruly but some lessons stuck. I ran away and defied my parents as any teen may do. I did not, however, get deeply entrenched in the world of drugs. I am thankful for the healthy fear that my parents instilled in me that kept me away from the drug scene. That is not to say that I was in the dark about drugs. Many of my friends were using and it was available to me at anytime but I chose to remain straight.

As I said earlier, I dated the kind of boys that most parents dread their daughters to bring home. I was enamored with my best friend in high school. We finally started to date but that was disastrous. It is true what they say about dating a friend. The friendship does not last after the breakup. I wonder whatever happened to him.

When I did agree to go on a date with someone my parents would approve of, that too turned out to be disastrous. He was not such a gentleman as he portrayed in front of others. He was also my brother's best friend, so I knew I would continue to have to face him again and again. I did see him again years later and he turned out to be a nice guy and the father of two beautiful children.

Beyond being in fear of the type of guys I dated I know now that the greater concern faced by my mother was the fear that if I had an asthma attack, who would do the right thing. Would someone else understand the severity of the situation? Would someone else understand the history and be able to communicate with the doctors? Would someone else be able to handle the situation and care for me the way she could? This was all more than my adolescent mind could handle. I had no clue. I would learn after I grew up and had children of my own.

Chapter 2

I grew up quickly. At least I thought I was grown up. By age twenty-five I was married with five children. My daughter was born in December of the year I graduated high school. My first son was born two and a half years later. I met a wonderful man who wanted to be with me and my two children. He wanted to share my life, even as chaotic as it seemed. Within three years we had another son. Then 362 days later, twin boys. We had a houseful. We moved to a house that needed work but was suitable for all of us. We decided to improve our lives through education. We both went to college at the same time. He earned an associate degree and I earned a bachelor's degree. I became a nurse.

The year I graduated from college was the same year the landlord decided to sell the house. He gave us a thirty-day notice to buy the house or move out. We opted to buy it. We believed it would be our "starter home" before moving on to a bigger and better house. Throughout this time, I had random asthma attacks. My husband was by my side through them all. He made the late-night drives to the emergency room. He took care of the family when I was hospitalized and continued working to keep money coming in. The attacks that I had seemed to be far fewer than the ones I had when I was growing up. It seemed that pregnancy and motherhood were good for my health.

It has been noted that stress affects asthma. The more the stress, the more likely an attack. But this was not terribly evident for me. As a young mother, a nursing student, a wife, and a member of a relatively poor family, my attacks were sparse by comparison. We faced hard times with so many children and so limited an education before my husband and I went back to school. We once received a turkey and all the fixings for Thanksgiving in a basket on our doorstep. We were the project family for the church. I know that was never in my plans as I am sure it was not what my parents had planned for me either. We often went to my in-laws' house for meals and were given any leftover and also extra food items to take home. I was now the one driving the beat-up old car.

Other stresses occurred as well during those years. My grandfather died the day I moved out of my parents' home. My grandmother died when I was five months pregnant. I was all registered to attend college right after high school. My mother and I did some serious head butting to the point of almost five years of silence. My husband and I found that little money, many children, and lack of maturity were a bad combination. We fought almost constantly. We tried counseling, but were both too young and too wrapped up in our own point of view to even learn how to communicate without blaming. Our oldest son experienced anaphylaxis with an unknown cause. Our daughter married a man we were certain was not the one for her. We knew, as parents, she would not be happy with her choice. Our second son accidentally stabbed himself while playing with a knife, and the social services got involved due to the nature of his injury. The twins were subjected to the daily drama and stress of being the youngest and of being teenage boys.

Eventually, the marriage fell apart. The two oldest children went with me and the three younger boys stayed with their father. We battled. We talked. We battled some more and then talked some more. Looking back I see that we never really separated our lives. We were friends whether we admitted it or not. Oh yes, we dated others. It should have been a clue but it took us seven years of being separated before we contacted attorneys and finally got divorced. So after eight years apart I am not sure if anyone, besides my ex-husband and I, was surprised that we moved back in together and remarried shortly thereafter. We were able to successfully reunite our family. Not everyone gets a second chance at perfection but we did. We took that chance and have been thankful for it every day since.

That was about the time when everything started falling apart. I received a call from my mother asking about the implications of some blood work results for my brother. He was sick and we were trying to second-guess the results before the doctors even knew what was going on. It turned out that my brother had cancer. This news was shocking in and of itself but even more so if you knew my brother. He was an athlete. He played soccer for thirty years. He was also a health nut. He ate fresh fruit every day. He exercised and worked hard. He even refused to use deodorant as it was a possible carcinogen. Of all people to have cancer, he seemed most unlikely.

Here I was, a mother of five who didn't exercise. An asthmatic who smoked almost a pack a day despite the hurt it caused my parents. I drank, not too excess but even so. And yet my brother gets cancer. He was given six months to a year to live. He lasted two years. During those two years I learned a lot about life from him. He surrounded himself with people that made him feel good about himself. He believed life was too short to be among people that make you feel bad. He continued to care about the condition of others. He wanted everyone in his life to be happy. He spent his adult years working with and as a fundraiser for children with terminal illnesses. His family and friends watched him slowly waste away, eaten by the cancer. He died, when he was forty-one years old, with his family and close friends at his side. He was an inspiration to so many. He was an inspiration to me.

It was during this time that my mother would later recall that I began complaining of vague stomach pain. I wrote it off as stress and barely recall complaining at the time. Just prior to the death of my brother my eczema, which I had since childhood, took a drastic change for the worse. Here my health problems started. From here I learned how inept and frightening our health care system is. Thus began a journey few would believe. But you just can't make up stuff like this.

Chapter 3

As a nurse, I placed a tremendous amount of faith in the health care system. I truly believed it was there to help people overcome illness or accept chronic illness, even death, with dignity. I knew that the system was there to help, not harm. I was proud to be a part of that system. I had seen it work. That system turned its head into an ugly beast as I faced challenging health issues. The system that I believed in was not true to my conviction.

I believe my calling into the realm of nursing began when I was a toddler. All those trips to the emergency room. All those admissions into the hospital. All the nurses who came to care for me. I saw and felt the care that was given. The nurses were dedicated, nurturing, and always there. I was afraid and they sat with me. They talked to me as if I were the only patient there. Even as a stubborn angry teenager, the nurses were still there to care for me. They never wrote me off as a waste of their time. They apologized if the treatment was going to hurt. They never lied and told me that it wouldn't hurt. Many times I needed blood work called arterial blood gases. This blood draw was unusually painful. The blood needed to come from an artery, not a vein, and the artery used is in the wrist. The needle is inserted and then wiggled a bit until the artery is penetrated. Often I would be bruised and swollen after the blood draw. But the nurses told me it would hurt. They told me it was okay to cry, even adults would cry. They told me how brave and strong I was. They made it all okay. When I was struggling to breathe they never left my side. They were there encouraging me to fight and letting me know it was okay to be scared. And I was scared.

When I decided to become a nurse I thought I had found my calling. I believed I was going down the altruistic path of giving to others what had been given to me. Early on in my career, I found psychiatric nursing. Helping to heal broken minds and broken spirits. I loved my work. I looked forward to going to work and caring for people of all ages, from three to one hundred and three, who were struggling with issues of the mind and heart. But the world of psychiatry was one with little funding and even less understanding from the general public. Each job was like walking a tightrope between patient care and wondering if the facility will be open the next day. Every state and federal budget cut claimed a facility or program. Resources for care dwindled and paychecks bounced. After several years of this, it was time to move on. I needed a job where the company was stable and the responsibilities allowed for expanding minds and offerings of hope. I became a teacher.

Teaching was an experience I will never forget. It was exciting and scary. It combined all the psychiatric skills I learned, all the emotional content of being part of a family, and all the dreams of so many students enmeshed into one classroom. It challenged my knowledge base, my nursing skills, my people skills, my organizational skills, and my communication skills. I was challenged to know more and do more so that each student received the best

I could give. The goal was to produce a nurse, but not just any nurse, a highly skilled and competent nurse.

At first I worked for a small private school. The classes were small and the atmosphere was one of friendly cooperative coworkers all sharing the same goal. There were stressful days too, though. It certainly was not all peaches and cream. The students argued, cried, complained, and sometimes just did not want to learn. There were students who failed out, but any teacher knew they had the heart to be a good nurse. Those days we cried to each other. We fought for supplies and resources. There was the expert dance of compromise that took place each time the program needed something extra. We did not always get what we wanted but we always managed. We had great graduating classes and we maintained our goal of producing highly competent nurses. Then it changed.

The corporate monster moved into town and bought the small private school. Many things changed. We were caught in the quagmire that is corporate America. Directives came from the left and right often without warning. And as far as corporations go, this one needed some serious communication education. The right and left hand did not know what the other was doing. Goals changed, but not on paper. We faced each day of work as a battle to just maintain our heads above water. We fought for major issues like computerized manikins and small items like paper. There was neither reason nor rhyme to the daily battles. And yet we continued on. The classes got bigger and bigger with more diversity in the classroom then one instructor could handle at a time. When we crossed paths in the hallway, we no longer smiled and said hello; we simply shook our heads and sighed, each knowing what was meant. There were still benefits though that kept each of us there. We got out of work each day at a reasonable time, no weekends, no holidays, and no mandated overtime. It was a gig of give and take. But when I became ill it began taking too much. Not only just because of the job itself but because of the energy I needed to maneuver through the dark and uncaring world of health care today.

Chapter 4

This dark and frightening journey started just before the death of my brother. My eczema started getting worse. At first I chalked it up to stress but it quickly became apparent that this was more than just stress. I contacted my allergist who prescribed prednisone and antibiotics. This proved to be a short-term answer and thus the pattern began. Large doses of prednisone with multiple course of antibiotics. The side effects of the prednisone took their toll. I developed a large round face due to fluid accumulation. I was susceptible to any bacteria out there as the prednisone suppressed my immune system. This continued for about eighteen months. I saw a local dermatologist who told me not to take hot showers, take oatmeal baths, and eat more dairy products. I continued to get worse. I later found out that I was allergic to oatmeal. I received a referral to a dermatology specialist in Boston.

When my mother and I got to Boston we were hopeful for some answers. This was not the first and only time we would be let down. In the exam room there were trays of vials for allergy testing. The doctor entered the room and spoke but she would not look at me. She stared at my arm throughout the exam. She said she needed to do allergy testing on me as I clearly had a "little rash" and proceeded to look for a clear patch of skin. At this point in time I had eczema on all skin surfaces except my face. I was bleeding and raw. I was holding fluids and my skin would weep with even the most gentle of touch. I told her I have no clear area, though she did not do any examination herself. She questioned if my feet were clear and I again let her know that I had no clear area of skin. She had planned to test me against 150 different allergens but I guess I ruined her plan by having eczema everywhere. She said she could do nothing for me since she could not perform the allergy testing. My mother, who sat quietly up to this point, then asked, "What about the edema?" as I was swollen with fluid. The doctor looked at her and snidely said, "Are you a nurse too?" I guess only nurses are supposed to be familiar with the term *edema*. We questioned the presence of an autoimmune disorder, and she looked at my arm and said, "You do not have an autoimmune disorder as you do not have the butterfly rash on your face." Again I became suspicious of her abilities as even I knew that there are more autoimmune disorders then the one that presents with a hallmark butterfly rash. That particular disorder is Lupus and, generally speaking, 35 percent of all cases do not even have the butterfly rash. At least at this point, my mother and I can look back and laugh at the incompetence of that doctor.

So the eczema continued. All anybody could do was watch as the eczema worsened. My friends, many of whom were nurses, were horrified with the health care system already. I wore long sleeves and turtlenecks to cover the disfiguring appearance of my skin. I made trips to the emergency room when I could no longer stand the pain and the itch. A doctor at the emergency room told me that he knew of patients that committed suicide due to the severity of the itch and the pain. This is not like poison ivy, even a severe case of poison ivy. It is ten times worse. With every movement my skin would tear and bleed. Each morning my night clothes were stained with blood from simply rolling over in my sleep. Every movement sent streaks of pain firing to my brain. Clothing was a pain inducing concept. Hot showers would relieve some of the itch but by hot I mean scalding. But of course, hot water was one of the worst things to do as it dries out the skin and makes the itch worse in the end. The emergency room doctor prescribed an antihistamine medication similar to Benadryl and told me to take as many as I needed in order to find some level of relief. I did. I was taking more than three times the normal dose. Yet I still went to work. My best friend, a seventeen-year veteran of acute care nursing, was astounded by the dosage I was told to take. It was quite a feat to just walk, let alone drive and function at work. I continued on the corticosteroids (prednisone) and antibiotics. My allergist was exasperated. He empathized for me but did not know what else to do as the severity of my condition was beyond his area of expertise. My next referral turned out much better.

The new dermatologist did a thorough exam. She could see that I was in a bad state. She said I was the second worse case she has seen in her many years as a dermatologist. She started me on a chemotherapy drug and photo treatments. The photo treatments consisted of twice weekly visits to the doctor's office. I would strip down to my under wear, step into a large tube and the therapy would begin. The tube was lined with lights. The lights would go on for a preset amount of time and essentially cook my skin. It was like being in a giant toaster. I would have to vacuum the base of the tube when I was done to clean up the dry dead skin that came off during treatment. The chemotherapy drug was prescribed at a lower dose than that of someone with cancer but it still had side effects to be aware of. One major side effect was the promotion of hair growth. I have string straight hair and thought, how bad could that be? Never thought of things like leg hair and moustaches. But oddly enough, not only did I not experience this side effect, but about a year into the treatment all my hair fell out. The dermatologist did a biopsy of my scalp and determined that I had alopecia areata which simply means my hair may never come back, or it may come back and fall out again, or it may come back and never fall out again. It was anybody's guess. You got to love the certainty of health care. After all was said and done though, my skin was repaired and I had a nice tan. But at last the itch and pain were gone. I thought it was over and I could be me again. Not so.

It only makes sense that since asthma and eczema go hand in hand, when one healed the other would exacerbate. And it did so with a vengeance. My asthma started kicking in almost daily. If you are unaware of what asthma is like, I will try to explain. Imagine if you can, having a plastic bag over your head with an elephant sitting on your chest. You are doomed. The elephant can be a baby or a fully grown adult. You cannot get air into your lungs. You cannot expand your lungs. Your muscles all hurt, especially in your back, as you continue the struggle to remain alive. It truly is a desperate terrifying experience. As a child, you do not know what is going on. As an adult, you understand but are still somewhat in the dark. As an adult and a nurse, you know exactly what is happening and what comes next.

In the past I knew my triggers. I could feel the attacks coming. I knew when to call the doctor and when to go to the emergency room. But that all changed. One day I was sitting on the couch watching a movie with my family. I walked to the kitchen and dropped to my knees. I couldn't breathe. I got to my bedroom and started taking my nebulizer treatment. This is a machine that vaporizes medication for rapid inhalation and absorption. It is meant for rapid relief of constriction of the airway. It did not work. For the first time since I was a young teenager I needed an ambulance. My children were scared and confused. My husband was terrified. One of my sons was at a friend's house one street away at the time. He was able to see the front of our house from where he was and saw the ambulance lights. Instead of taking the time to get into his car and come home, he simply jumped a six-foot fence and ran home. Needless to say this was new experience for the whole family.

This continued on and on for months. There were multiple speed runs to the emergency room including the one time we actually had to go to the nearest fire department for an ambulance as we were not going to make it to the emergency room in time. There were multiple admissions with multiple consults regarding this new change in my asthma symptoms. A new doctor was brought on board and after a few visits with him a suggestion was made that this maybe an autoimmune disorder called Churg-Strauss. This statement was the fuel for everything that came next.

But in the meantime at the end of one hospital admission for an asthma attack I experienced yet another problem. On the day I was to be discharged as I was changing out of the hospital Johnny and into my own clothes for the trip home, I started vomiting. It was violent and fast and it was bile. I called the nurse and in a whirlwind I was assessed by a surgeon. I was scheduled for surgery the next morning. So much for the anticipated discharge. The surgeon stated that I had a "hot" gallbladder and it needed to come out. I went through the surgery successfully and without complication. I was discharged forty-eight hours later.

I was referred to a local rheumatologist to explore the concept of this autoimmune disorder, Churg-Strauss. This doctor stated he did not think that was the issue but ran some blood work anyhow. He also decided to test for hepatitis B and hepatitis A exposure as I am a health care worker. The hepatitis C came back positive. Now the downward spiral began and the hepatitis seemed to become the basis for all future assessments, recommendations, and treatment protocols.

I asked my primary care physician for a copy of my records and sent them to a large hospital in Maryland for review for a second opinion on the Churg-Strauss. They recommended a doctor in the Boston area. I asked my primary care physician for a referral and he stated that he thought I was being too concerned about this issue. He documented that I was belligerent and hostile. (I later found out he was under review by the American Medical Association for denying referrals.) I went to Boston anyway.

There the doctor had not read my records before my appointment. I guess two months isn't enough time for a record to be read. He read them in the exam room during the appointment while my husband and I waited for forty-five minutes. He also responded to five alerts from his beeper. He then simply stated, "I do not think you have Churg-Strauss. You may have it but it is such a slow progressing illness. I just do not see it yet." And with that we went home. It was time to now focus on the hepatitis C.

Chapter 5

Hepatitis C is a viral infection that is passed through blood. Some people get it from a large blood exposure working in a health care environment. Not me. Some get it from a history of multiple sex partners, although this is the least likely form of transmission. Not me. Some get it from intravenous drug use and sharing needles. Not me. Others get it from a tattoo or body piercing where the equipment used is not sterile and is reused from one customer to the next. Not me. As luck would have it, more stringent guidelines were placed on tattoo and body-piercing establishments so that equipment sharing is not allowed. The industry, though, seems to have found a loophole. They use clean, sterile equipment but they reuse ink. This way they do not have to incur more cost by opening fresh ink for every customer. How clever. But apparently the end result can be the same. It seems this is where I acquired hepatitis C. One little tattoo from a certified establishment in trade for a lifetime of worry.

Hepatitis C usually attacks the liver causing cirrhosis and sometimes liver cancer. This concept scared me as there is a long history of cancer in our family, and cancer killed my brother a little over a year prior to my diagnosis. Off to the doctor I went.

The doctor that specializes in this is usually a gastroenterologist although there are also infectious disease specialists and hepatologists (liver specialists). I chose a gastroenterologist. The doctor told me that my viral count was "significantly" elevated and I needed to start treatment immediately. The treatment basically consisted of injecting poison and taking some poison pills. The injection is called interferon and it is often given weekly. The pills are antivirals and they are taken daily. This drug combination has some potentially serious side effects that can preclude an individual from completing the treatment. The treatment is generally a forty-eight-week ordeal. This time frame can vary depending on the type of hepatitis C one has. I heeded the doctor's message and started the treatment right away. Let the games begin.

The first injection was done by the doctor, and the rest were to be done by my husband (after I taught him how). I immediately felt the effects. I was tired and lethargic. I quickly became more and more of a lump on my couch than an active adult. I continued to work although I knew my performance was altered but one needs an income. In about a month I started getting stomach pain. It quickly worsened and I responded by eating less. The pain intensified every time I ate, no matter what I ate or how much. One call to the doctor and they let me know that a complication of the treatment was pancreatitis, a painful infection of the pancreas. Blood work would confirm or disprove this diagnosis. For me, no pancreatitis. This was a good thing but yet the pain continued. The doctor, for whatever reason, decided it did not warrant further investigation as he believed the pain was not related to the treatment or the virus. Remember though, he is a gastroenterologist who deals with all issues of the gastric system, from mouth to anus. I was losing weight rapidly and getting weaker week by week. Everyone around me, family and friends, became concerned. At one appointment with the doctor, my husband asked, "How much weight loss is acceptable before stopping the treatment?" The doctor replied that the treatment does not get stopped until the patient stops it. They recommend staying on the treatment as long as the patient can take it. They also said that stopping and restarting the treatment at a different time would be detrimental as the second round would be less effective because the virus could develop defenses to the treatment once exposed to it. Clever virus. I did stop the treatment, though, after twenty-two weeks. I had lost forty pounds and could no longer go on. I had a little extra weight to lose anyhow at the onset of this treatment, but 110 pounds and a height of 5'4", I found it unacceptable. At that point my body was breaking down the muscle mass just for survival. But on the upside, my asthma was greatly improved.

After stopping the treatment, the pain subsided a bit. It did not go away but became more tolerable. I was able to increase my nutritional intake and actually gain a few pounds. Six months after stopping the treatment my blood was checked again for the virus. The doctor phoned to say the count was high again. He recommended that I go back on the treatment but if I could not commit to the full forty-eight weeks then there was no point. I thought that statement was a little harsh, coming from a professional in a caring profession. I explained that the stomach pain was still there and at this point had been increasing. Again he focused on the need to start the treatment and blatantly ignored my concern about the stomach pain. It was time for a new doctor.

Now my head was spinning. I had suffered through the loss of my brother, the devastation that event caused to the rest of my family, the exacerbation of the eczema, the exacerbation of the asthma, feeling shunned by my primary care, my gastroenterologist, and the specialist in Boston. Could this really be a streak of bad luck? I started questioning myself and what I was doing wrong. I could not fathom why I the medical system was not paying attention. Maybe I just wasn't sick enough. I believe the health care system has become so focused on trauma and devastatingly acute illness that anything less is seen as whining. I just could not believe how inept and bungling the system had become. But I was in for a greater shock as this process continued to spiral out of control.

I went to the new gastroenterologist with hope. I was seeking answers that I believed he had. The doctor took the time to listen to my medical history and the cause for my concern. He scheduled an endoscopy later in the month. An endoscopy is a test where they insert a tube with a tiny camera on the end, down your throat and into the gastrointestinal tract. Through this device they can also take tissue samples for biopsy. I thought that this doctor was going to take me seriously and achieve a goal of determining the cause of my pain. I was truly hopeful. He also scheduled a CT scan which takes pictures of your insides almost like an X-ray but far more detailed. Now we are going to get somewhere.

The endoscopy and CT scan came back normal. Well, this is good. It can't be anything really bad if these two tests did not find it. The doctor then said he thought it might be just a spasm issue where the intestinal tract is not synchronizing its movements. The movement of the intestinal tract is called peristalsis. He started me on a medication to help the process of peristalsis. After one single dose the pain went away. Voila, he found the answer. I was overjoyed. After three doses I could not see clearly. Not because of the joy but because of a side effect of the medication. I was at work but could only see from the very edges of my peripheral vision. So much for driving the thirty-five-mile trip home. My husband had to come get me and have our son drive my truck home. The doctor stopped the medication and I was better in about forty-eight hours. I was glad to have my vision back but now what? The pain was back. Does it really need to be a trade-off between the pain and my ability to see? How unfair is this?

The doctor started me on a new medication that is supposed to aid in peristalsis but told me from the start that it is less effective. He was right. Actually it was not less effective; it had no effect at all. He added an anti-depressant as some anti-depressants have an added benefit of relieving nerve pain. The downside was that it takes two to four weeks to build up to a therapeutic level in the body. Okay then, I was ready to face another month of pain. Maybe at the end of that time there would be relief especially since I was losing two to four pounds a week. I know every woman seems to want to lose weight but this is not the diet plan anyone has in mind. People around me were starting to notice the change. Some people at my job stopped making eye contact. They could see that this was not just some diet. They saw that this was an illness. Some were bold enough to ask. One man, who I spoke with on occasions when our departments crossed paths, actually walked into my office and simply asked, "Are you sick?" No salutations, no pleasantries, just a single question. At least no one can say men are subtle and mystifying.

I went to my primary care physician for help. She proceeded to come in the room with the wrong patient chart. Then she wrote a prescription with the wrong patient name. She told me to drink fifteen milliliters two times a day and the prescription actually read take one tablet twice a day. I chalked this up to her having a bad day. I truly could not wrap my head around the idea that a doctor could be that incompetent and still be in a practice.

As time went on and the medication did not work, again I grew weaker each day. My frustration, anger, and determination were the fuel that I ran on to get through each day. Finally, the pain reached a breaking point. I left work in the morning. I called the gastroenterologist on my way home and his nurse took down my information and concern. She phoned me back saying, "The doctor said there is nothing more he can do for you, so go to the emergency room if you are really in that much pain."

As a nurse, I found this reaction to my call rather upsetting. I saw it as a waste of medical resources especially since the emergency room would try to relieve the pain and then refer me out to a gastroenterologist. As a patient in pain, I was devastated. Here I was shunned again. Somehow, I was not deserving enough for even the slightest bit of attention from a physician. This lack of care became the pivotal moment when I started believing in the biased distribution of care. I began reflecting on the cause of this bias. Then it came to me. Maybe I was being shunned because I was hepatitis C positive and seen as seeking pain medication. This combination made me a target for stereotyping as a drug user and not worthy of care by mainstream medicine. As a psychiatric nurse this thought was nauseating.

I pondered, cried, fumed, and vented to anyone that would listen, usually my husband, my mother, or my two best friends. My husband spent each day reading calorie and nutrition books trying to plan a meal for me. He would prepare foods with the most impact in the smallest portions. He would give me a blueberry muffin, or a peanut butter and jelly sandwich each morning. I would take it to work and my goal was to eat the muffin or sandwich before I left work to come home. I had eight hours to eat and often did not meet the goal. My friends would come into my office and jokingly, gently point out the lack of bites taken from the food. They too were monitoring my intake. It was absurd and almost comical if it weren't so serious. I seemed to have been stuck in a cycle of bias and disdain. I worked with nurses all day as the manager of a nursing program. No one could understand the illogic and lack of urgency the medical world was displaying. I went back to my primary care physician to see if there were other options. This time I was hit full force with the bias I had previously thought was present. Now I knew it to be true.

For this appointment, my primary care doctor phoned the gastroenterologist and reported back to me that the gastroenterologist did not feel that I needed pain medication. Therefore my primary care would not prescribe any. I asked her what else I was supposed to do as I was slowly starving to death. She rolled her eyes and said, "Oh, give me a break." She then offered to refer me to a nutritionist and I promptly asked for her rationale for this referral. She said that the nutritionist would help me make better food choices. I was now angry and offended. I asked the doctor if the nutritionist would prescribe an ointment for providing essential nutrients via osmosis as my food choices were not the issue. Pain was the issue. My doctor then proceeded to tell me that some people have pain for no reason. The nurse in me shot back that just because the medical world could not find the cause does not mean that there is no reason. Nor does it mean that one should stop looking for the cause. Her next statement showed her true colors as a "professional." She looked at me and said, "Give me a break. It is not my fault that you do not feel well." Then she told me that I was being abusive to her and she did not need to be my doctor. Quite frankly she should probably not be anyone's doctor. She then told me that if pain was the issue I should go to the emergency room for help. Unbelievable, another doctor passing the buck. I was stunned but this time I did go to the emergency room. I was given medication for the pain and a referral to a gastroenterologist. I was not surprised by this course of treatment.

So there I was left in pain, no answers, nowhere to turn to, and still in need of treatment for the hepatitis C. I opted to go to an infectious disease specialist and start round two of the treatment of interferon and the antiviral medication. I was determined and ready. I was not going to risk the chance of liver cancer with the extensive cancer history in my family. As the treatment began, I continued to try to manage the stomach pain and find some help. I explained to the infectious disease specialist the issue I was having with abdominal pain. She was concerned and tried to do all she could while I continued seeking help and a determination of the cause of the pain. She did all she could, which was prescribe pain medication so I could tolerate small amounts of food, but gastroenterology was not her area of practice. She was sympathetic but limited in options to help me.

Chapter 6

My mother lives close to me but in a different state. She recommended that I try a bigger hospital in her state in the hope that they will be more progressive and aware than the doctors I had dealt with up to this point. My closest friend also used to work at this particular hospital and she agreed that was probably my next best course of action. I made an appointment. I tried very hard to fight the "here we go again" thoughts that were clogging my brain. I tried to go with a positive attitude. I tried but did not succeed.

The doctor took her time with me. She listened closely. She asked questions. She did her assessment. I now weighed 108 pounds. She thoughtfully prepared a response to me, my husband, and my parents. She said that clearly I needed help and that I needed an answer. She said that my weight was dangerously low and that she would stick by me until an answer was found. She asked me if I was open to the idea of alternate feeding via a G-tube. This is a tube placed through the abdomen and directly into the stomach and feeding is done through the tube. She asked about the interferon treatment but did not focus on it. She suggested that I stop the treatment again as it might be exacerbating the problem. I told her that I would consider it but that the treatment was working and that I did not want to take a chance unless it really was the cause of the pain. She agreed that it was not causing the pain. As we left the appointment, I believe I heard a collective sigh of relief. There was hope again. This doctor was serious and she was going to help me. What a good feeling. This doctor was going to schedule the testing and collaborate with her peers for an answer. She initiated the reaffirmation of trust in the medical world.

Then days went by and no appointments for testing were happening. I kept calling the doctor and asking why. I was given the run around by whoever answered the phone. Finally, after three weeks, she scheduled a CTA. This is a CT scan that looks specifically at the vascular structures. Then my next appointment with her happened and I was once again reeling. She came into the exam room ninety minutes late. Not a good start. This time she did not even bring my chart into the room. She said that the CTA was fine and then asked if I had stopped the interferon. I told her that I did not. She then told me that the interferon must be causing the pain and that if I did not stop it then there was nothing she could do. My husband and mother had many questions for her. As they were asking their questions, the doctor stated that she needed to attend to her other patients as they were getting upset by the lengthy wait. We were brushed off, again. But out of that we did get a referral to Johns Hopkins, and I sent my records there and requested a review as no doctor could not, yet, definitively rule out Churg-Strauss. Abdominal pain, worsening asthma, and eczema exacerbations are all symptoms of Churg-Strauss but they could all be symptoms of something else as well. It was all so confusing. So many people were offering advice and information that it was hard to keep it all straight. Then there is the Internet as well. My husband certainly should have earned a medical degree through the research he was doing daily on the Internet.

The running joke in my family was always about the fact that I am not normal. By that I mean I have never really had the accepted normal symptoms of an illness. I did not fit in the medical model box. That only served to complicate the issue now. How can one decide what is wrong when the symptoms don't fit the way they are expected to?

Churg-Strauss is an uncommon autoimmune disorder. One hallmark of this disorder is asthma. Not everyone who has asthma will develop Churg-Strauss but everyone with Churg-Strauss has asthma. Usually an indicator is the worsening of asthma symptoms. The real clincher, though, is a high eosinophil count. Eosinophils are one type of white blood cell. These eosinophils can accumulate in any organ affected as Churg-Strauss is a vascular disorder. So anywhere the blood goes, so do the eosinophils. The percentage of eosinophils in the affected organ is the giveaway for Churg-Strauss. But my eosinophil count did not climb high enough. The other hallmarks were in place but the count wasn't quite high enough. But then again the treatment for the hepatitis C will decrease the eosinophil count, so the test could have been inaccurate. I know this is all very confusing but this was the hand I was dealt. This was my daily life.

Then the phone call came. Johns Hopkins wanted to see me. They did not refer me to another doctor in my area but they said they wanted to see me. I made the appointment. Hope anew. I struggled through the next month. Hopeful anticipation. Fear of the answer but needing an answer. Growing weaker and thinner by the day. I was below one hundred pounds. I was starving, though

I no longer felt the actual pangs of hunger. We planned the trip to Baltimore, Maryland. My parents came with my husband and me. We scheduled the time off from our jobs, bid farewell to friends, and boarded the train for a six-hour ride early in the morning the day before my appointment. We traveled with well wishes from friends and family.

It seems odd that after all I have been through that I could even remotely experience hope anymore but I did. It was cautious hope but it was still there. I guess when you give up hope you give up everything. I could not and would not do that. You see I am, what is commonly referred to as, a control freak. I like being in charge. I like having control over myself and my environment. I am not a power hungry jerk but simply someone who likes order and logic. I accept challenges and am willing to take some chances. My expectations of others are the same as those for myself: do the job to the best of one's abilities, do not play mind games with others, be fair, and laugh at yourself. I also do not give up easily. If I believe there is an answer or resolution to be found then I will continue looking. I believe in standing tall, standing up, and holding true to one's convictions. This may sound very cliché but there are still some of us out there who live by these standards. I am one.

Prior to the pain I was an active adult. My husband referred to me as the energizer wife because it seemed I never stopped. If something needed to be done, then do it. Now, since the pain, I have been forced to become a different person. I am a slave to the pain every moment of every day. I spend my time in bed, hands clenched, not moving. It breaks my heart that my three-year-old granddaughter's memories of this time with her grandmother will consist of climbing on my bed, snuggling, and watching television.

We should be outside playing, riding her bike, making mud pies, but instead she snuggled because I could not do those things with her. At the age of three her concept of health care is very simple, kiss the boo-boo. She asked everyday, "Mama (she could not pronounce grandma), does your belly hurt?" This boo-boo could not be kissed away.

So I was able to still find hope in the trip we were now on. After all I was going to Johns Hopkins. This is a large world-renown hospital and medical center. Surely they would be able to help me. My husband, mother, and father all clung to hope as well. We rode mostly in silence, each lost in their thoughts and fears. Each of us looked at this from a different perspective. My parents had already lost a son to cancer. The fear of losing a daughter to unknown abdominal pain and starvation was unthinkable. My husband was watching his wife suffer. He saw me in pain everyday. He saw the weight loss, the weakness, the frustration, and tears. He saw it all and was helpless. There was nothing he could do to help me. He also kept secure in his heart the thoughts that we had been apart already for eight years and we reunited and rekindled our love; he did not want to lose me again. For him this fear crossed every action and every thought every day.

For me, I closed my eyes and worried that this would be my last chance. I had no plan of what could be next if Johns Hopkins could not help. But mostly I spent my time pushing that thought out of my head.

Chapter 7

Johns Hopkins. Now we are in the big league. The medical center campus is huge. I feel so humbled just driving into the campus. And this was just one of the many. Apparently, Johns Hopkins is spread out within the Baltimore limits. My appointment was set with a doctor in the respiratory center. I was first seen by the fellow, not a man but a doctor in training, in the office. She was thorough and quiet. She completed a full assessment and history. She asked questions and documented the answers. Then she left the room. Nothing impressive so far. Then the doctor came in.

The doctor was open, friendly, and down to earth. As he spoke I realized he did not see me as the others saw me. He spoke to me as a patient. I was not a nurse. I was not an annoyance. I was not hepatitis C. I was not an unknown abdominal pain. I was a person. I was someone in need of help. I needed his help. He was there to help me. He delivered the message that he did not feel my symptoms were that of Churg-Strauss. But he did not stop there. He did not just brush me off telling me what I did not have but talked about what he thought the problem was even though it was outside his specialty. He stepped outside his comfort zone to help me. Now I was impressed. Here was a doctor that took his job seriously and took patient care seriously. He believed my problem was a spasm or increased pressure in the sphincter of Oddi. This sphincter aids in moving food from the stomach to the intestines where absorption of nutrients occurs and waste is separated. Correction of this problem maybe as simple as cutting a slit in the sphincter to decrease the pressure.

This doctor then referred me to a colleague of his at a hospital across town. The colleague was a gastrointestinal specialist. The doctor at Johns Hopkins promised to talk to his colleague and see if anything could be done before I had to leave Baltimore and go back home. So I went back to the hotel room to wait but this time there was a single candle of hope to light the way.

We waited for twenty-four hours; then I called the office of the new doctor. His secretary phoned me back with an appointment for two days later. She scheduled the procedure to fix the sphincter of Oddi. All she needed from me was insurance data and medical records. I let her know that the doctor at Johns Hopkins had all the records and she agreed to call for a copy. I called as well to authorize and confirm the transmission of the records. I knew this may not be an easy task as my records contained approximately 200 pages of notes and lab test results from four doctors spanning four years. We enjoyed the next day as a family.

We went out to see the sites of Baltimore. I was in a wheelchair at this time as I did not have the energy to walk. I had grown too weak to sightsee. But we were able to tour the harbor shops and go to the aquarium. It was such a nice treat to feel the relief of the upcoming resolution. The pain was now tolerable only due to the psychological relief. The procedure was scheduled for noon the next day.

It was a Friday and the sun was shining. There was a little crisp bite in the air as it was autumn. I cried. I cried all morning. I could not stop the tears from coming. I could not even grasp the magnitude of what was about to happen. I was scared and joyful at the same time. I was not going to be in pain any more. After one and a half years of abdominal pain, it was finally going to end. I was thinking of all the foods I would be able to eat. I couldn't decide what I would eat first. I had been craving spaghetti and hot sausage for what seemed like forever. This is my favorite meal. But as it was autumn it was time for the pumpkin muffins at Dunkin Donuts. They are such a special treat. But there I sat in the wheelchair with the sun on my face, crying. I had absolutely no control over the tears. But at last it was time to get into the taxi and go to the hospital.

Chapter 8

I was cold. Shivering. I was in pain. Pain medication was not allowed twenty-four hours prior to the procedure. The registration process was amazingly quick and easy. I was now in the prep room and the nurse came in to complete the pre-procedure assessment. She brought three heated blankets with her. She was a goddess as far as I was concerned. There were a lot of other patients there, too, in various states of consciousness. Some were being prepped as I was. Some had just come back from having their procedure done. And some were waiting on discharge. They were here for so many reasons as this room had patients getting ready for any number of gastrointestinal procedures. The IV was now in my arm and I just needed to wait for the doctor to call for me. The countdown to pain-free living was streaming in my head. My husband and mother were there with me and they were even joking around as we waited. My dad was back at the hotel awaiting the call that the procedure was done and all went well.

The doctor stepped into the area where I was. He came over and I was anticipating the usual greeting and introduction. Then he should explain the procedure to me and off we go. But that did not happen. He came over and gruffly stated his name, and then asked me why I was there. He didn't know who I was or why I was there. I told him about Johns Hopkins and the possible problem with my sphincter of Oddi. I told him about speaking with his secretary and about the records at Johns Hopkins. He said that he received no records. He went on to say that the procedure I was scheduled for was very risky and could have serious complications. He said that he could not and would not perform this procedure as I was not strong enough for it, and he didn't even know me or my history. He needed to review my records first. And he left. And I cried.

All the hustle and bustle of the room was still happening. Other patients were coming in to prep. Some moved out for their procedure and others went home. I did not see or hear any of this. I was lost. I was stunned. Not again! Why me? Is there any chance I will ever feel better?

The doctor came back in the room and told us that he did not have any records. They were never sent from Johns Hopkins. He called over to Johns Hopkins to get them but was told that my records were sent to the medical records department already and therefore unobtainable as they were in limbo. He also could not get in touch with his secretary to have her track them down. He asked if I had another copy with me. Really? No, I did not. I had the originals at home but that was six hours away, one way. So we did the next best thing. We called our son at home and had him bring the two-hundred page record to the nearest Staples store to have them faxed.

Faxing records requires that it get scanned into a computer first and then sent. We were stunned when our son called back to say that there was a service fee and faxing would cost one dollar and fifty cents per page. This would cost over three hundred dollars to send. So we opted to use e-mail; we just needed an e-mail address to send to. We tried to contact the doctor's office, as he was in doing another procedure on a different patient while awaiting the records. We were hoping his secretary would be available. No luck. No doctor and no answer at his office left us with no e-mail address. Each of us wanted to scream. But that would not have been the appropriate way to convey frustration in the middle of the prep room. So we continued to try to reach the doctor's secretary. At long last, the nurse on the unit who was witnessing this mess offered her personal e-mail address so that we could get the records. Another goddess to the rescue. Finally the records came through. They were printed and handed over to the doctor. He went away to read and review. We waited. And waited. And waited.

He came back with the knowledge of me and my history in his head. He asked for me to explain my history and chronicle the course of care and testing I had already been through. He listened. I don't mean he heard what I said; I mean he listened. He took brief notes and asked for clarification as needed. He then said that if I were from the area he would simply schedule an office appointment and start this process over. But he could not do that for two very important reasons. One, I was not from the area, and two, he saw that I was not strong enough or well enough to wait any longer. He clearly stated that I was acutely ill regarding the weight loss and something needed to be done quickly. He told me to come back to the hospital on Monday, and he would have me admitted for five days and run every test that he could. He did not play games, and he did not talk in circles or with vague or complicated medical jargon. He promised to look as hard as he could but did not promise resolution. Each test result would dictate what would come next, and by Friday of the following week, at the very least, we would know what the problem wasn't. So six hours after coming in to the hospital crying with hope, we left the hospital crying with frustration. We have been down this road before.

My dad could not stay with us for another week. His job would not allow it. So in the morning, despite the road closures due to the Baltimore marathon, he got in a cab and headed for the train station. He made it home shortly after dinner time and called at least twice a day from there through the following week. I missed him.

Chapter 9

At nine on Monday morning, I was being checked in at the hospital. I finally made it to a room by noon. The admitting nurse came in and completed her assessment. Ninety-five pounds, dressed. Dehydrated and weak but with admitting orders that I was to have nothing by mouth. Many of the tests the doctor was planning to do required a completely empty stomach. This would not be a problem. So the IV was started and fluids were entering my body through the vein in my arm. The only test scheduled for that day, though, was a CT scan, the test that is similar to an X-ray but more detailed. The next morning the invasive testing began. The phlebotomist came in to draw some blood. Phlebotomists are often lovingly referred to as vampires. Boy, this was never a truer statement. She came in apologizing. She said that she needed a lot of blood as the doctor ordered so many tests. She said that some of the tests he ordered she had never even heard of and had to look them up. She then inserted the needle and proceeded to take fifteen vials of blood. I was just glad I did not pass out from being drained of blood.

Later that morning the doctor performed an endoscopy whereby sending a camera down my throat and into my stomach via a tube. He took several tissue samples for biopsy along the way. Then, while still under anesthesia, he did a colonoscopy. A colonoscopy is basically the same as an endoscopy but it enters the body through the other end and looks at the portion of the gastrointestinal tract that could not be viewed from the endoscopy. The colonoscopy itself is not too bad because you sleep through it. Blissfully unaware. The difficult part of a colonoscopy is the prep. You need to be thoroughly cleaned out, so the doctor can get a good look at the intestines. In order to be cleaned out, you need to drink a cleansing fluid the night before. The average person needs to drink a lot in order for the full effect but since I have not eaten much in the last year or so, I got off easy. The nurse brought in the gallon of cleansing fluid. Ironically, it is called go-lightly. This fluid tastes like dirty water. You need to keep drinking until your stool becomes a clear liquid. Prior to a colonoscopy most people need to drink the whole gallon. My status allowed me to get away with drinking two glasses. After the procedure was completed, I visited with my family and then simply slept.

Well into the evening, a doctor came into my room. He said that he was referred to me to discuss hepatitis C as he is a hepatic specialist. This means he specializes in liver functions and liver disease.

When I originally started the hepatitis C treatment, my doctor at the time told me that my viral count was significantly high and stressed the importance of starting the treatment as soon as possible. So I did. When I was unable to complete the treatment and my viral count increased again, my new doctor was concerned. I was told that each time you start and stop the treatment, the virus can develop resistance to the treatment and, therefore, make each successive attempt less effective. So I started again, with the goal of eliminating this virus from my body.

The hepatic specialist came in to talk to me about the hepatitis C and the treatment. He was well known and an expert in this field. What he had to say surprised and stunned us all. He said everything opposite of what I had previously been told. He said that the viral count did not matter unless you are on the treatment and trying to determine the efficacy of it. Other than that it is just a number. When you have the virus you have the virus. A higher viral count does not mean you are more sick or more at risk for cirrhosis or liver cancer. He reviewed my liver biopsy results and noted, as the record did, that there was no damage to my liver now. His recommendation would have been to come in for a liver biopsy every three to five years to monitor for liver damage. If liver damage occurred then, and only then, would he initiate treatment. Some people can live with this virus their whole lives and never have a problem. Even if the virus causes damage, it can take decades to develop. Bottom line: I did not need to put myself through the treatment and the side effects at all. It was unnecessary to have done all this so soon. I may have been one of the ones who never developed a problem. But even if I did, it may not be until I am much older. It was essentially a colossal waste of time. This doctor then said with certainty that neither the treatment nor the virus was the cause of my pain. It just does not happen like that. He wished me luck with the testing to determine the cause of the pain and then said that he would like to follow up on my hepatitis status over the next few years. He asked me to call him after the cause of the pain was found.

After he left the room, my mom, husband, and I just stared at each other. We could not believe what we just heard. My faith in the health care system in the northeast was finally shaken to the core. We started talking about the information the hepatic specialist had given us. We made a final determination to stop the treatment once and for all. It was over and I would follow up with the hepatic specialist later. With the interferon and antiviral drugs leaving my system, maybe the lethargy will go away too.

The pain continued. I was scheduled for three more tests and allowed a clear liquid diet. This meant water, broth, Jell-O, but not red Jell-O, and clear or light-colored juices. This was fine with me as I had long since stopped feeling hunger. Any time I ate within the last eighteen months was merely because I had to and not because I wanted to. Outrageously salty hospital broth would be fine. It really did not matter to me.

The next day the testing was to continue but due to a scheduling error nothing happened. The day after that, an upper GI series was arranged. For this test one has to drink a substance similar to pop rocks. This substance creates gas and opens some of the gastrointestinal structures. Then you are given a thick chalky fluid to drink. You have to drink it quickly as the radiologist takes pictures of the fluid moving through the upper portion of the gastrointestinal tract. For me, I then needed to sit and wait while pictures were taken every half hour until the fluid entered my colon. This took six hours.

Lastly, on the final day in the hospital, I was taken to complete a gastric emptying study. For this study the patient eats an egg sandwich and drinks a little water. The egg sandwich is not the same as what one would get at McDonalds or Dunkin Donuts. Instead it is made of egg whites only. Then a radioactive material is added to the egg so the camera can follow the food. This test is used to determine how fast a person's stomach empties the food into the intestinal tract. For the average adult, the stomach should move the food out in four to six hours, depending on the size of the meal and the individual themselves.

So now all the testing was complete. The doctor did as promised. He tested me for everything he could in the time frame he had to work within. Some of the blood work had not come back yet as they could take several weeks to process. The upper GI series and the gastric emptying study results would not be ready for a couple days. Now the doctor concluded that I had functional bowel disorder. This is called an umbrella diagnosis which means that my gastrointestinal tract was not working correctly. This type of diagnosis is general, vague, and covers a wide area, hence the name umbrella diagnosis. It is tech talk for abdominal pain with no known source. It is tech talk for I don't know what is wrong. The doctor gave me two new prescriptions, one for the pain and the other for increasing the smoothness of peristalsis. He also asked that I call him at the end of the following week for a follow-up conversation. The next day we were on the train and heading home.

I was pleased to have had the million-dollar workup but disappointed with the result. I was thrilled that it was not something horrendous or fatal. I was hoping for something that could be fixed. I got an umbrella diagnosis with no plan to address the ongoing starvation or the pain besides pain medication. The medication that he prescribed for peristalsis was the same one I had been on in the past. It did not work then and I did not think it would work now.

Chapter 10

Back at home it felt great to be surrounded by our children and grandchildren. We missed them all so much while we were gone. But when the hugs, kisses, and phone calls to friends were done, reality set in.

I am ninety-five pounds on pain medication for an indeterminate time, no good plan for how to eat, a doctor six hours away, and not one good doctor in my hometown area to follow up with. I almost felt worse than what I had before we went to Baltimore. Nowhere to turn to. As I tried to wrap my brain around all this, I sulked for two days. Then the phone call came.

The doctor from Baltimore phoned to give me the results of the gastric emptying study. He told me that after one and a half hours, less than 10 percent of the food had passed out of my stomach and into the intestinal tract. This number was very far off from normal. I now had a reason for the pain and a true diagnosis: gastroparesis. Gastroparesis translates to paralyzed stomach. This all meant that the muscles in my stomach were not working anymore or just barely working. When I ate food, it sat in my stomach and did not get pushed into the intestinal tract by the muscles of the stomach. Then when I ate again, the new food pushed the old food out. But this was a painful process. The food sitting in my stomach basically rot and when it did move through there is very little, if any, nutrients left for absorption. Malnutrition became a huge issue with this disorder. The rest of the conversation with doctor consisted of a change in medication and an explanation of how to eat with a weight gain goal. He said he did not feel hopeful that the initial medication would be very effective but I needed to try it, and there was one serious side effect called tardive dyskinesia. Tardive dyskinesia means involuntary muscle movements that range from uncontrollable lip smacking to a complete freeze of all muscles. But he also told me of another medication that had more success. The problem with that medication is that it is not FDA approved. I could go online and order it through a Canadian pharmacy though. Neither of these pharmacological interventions sounded promising but they were certainly worth a try. It couldn't get much worse from where I currently am. Could it?

He said that my eating practices would need to change drastically. I would need to eat six to eight meals a day. These meals would have to be very small; essentially, I needed to truly eat like a bird. I had found two or three bites are all that can be handled at a time. I needed to avoid fat, fiber, chocolate, coffee, dairy products, any caffeinated drinks, and carbonated drinks. All fruits and vegetables needed to be cooked. Raw fruits and vegetables contain fiber that is too difficult to digest, so it needed to be cooked to initiate the breaking-down process. Also, since this disorder is unpredictable regarding the occurrence of pain, I needed to avoid any food that I found to cause pain. But foods that are fine one day may not be fine the next. I would need to muddle my way through my daily menu until I found something that worked for me, day by day. The doctor also set a lofty goal of a twenty-pound weight gain. He stated this goal with a lilt in his voice that told me this goal is not likely to occur and certainly not anytime soon.

I never once thought that putting on weight could be so difficult. People worry all their lives about putting on weight and they certainly do not want to listen to the struggles of someone who needs to but can't. Our society centers itself around food. Social events, holidays, bad days, and good days are all associated with food. Coping and celebrating are both done with food. Then society demands that people be thin and beautiful. Thin maybe nice but anorectic is not. When I saw myself in the mirror I saw skin and bones. My muscle mass had been worn down by my body breaking it down for nutrition. This look was far from healthy and even farther from sexy. It was more aptly representative of a POW than a supermodel. There is nothing beautiful about starvation.

This disorder is not rare. It is not uncommon but it is relatively unknown. The two gastroenterologists that I had seen in the past should have been able to test and diagnose this problem. There was no reason, except pure assumption, bias, and prejudice that I needed to suffer for several months beyond that which was necessary. Our medical system let me down. That which I believed in, dedicated my career to, and regarded with great pride, turned its back and left me to fend for myself. The medical system left me disillusioned, lost, angry, and almost hopeless. I now find myself in the throes of the internal conflict of my concept of nursing and health care, and the reality I was forced to face.

When looking at a struggle though, maybe, it is the change, rebirth if you will, that comes with struggle that is the silver lining.

When faced with challenges, our perspectives may change and in so doing, our view of the world and our lives change. Our priorities change and our concept of what is important changes, and that can only be good. Family and friends take priority over jobs and status. Money to live is more than enough instead of always trying to have money to play. In that change one can only hope is a sense of peace; a sense of coping. One knows when it is time to move on from the struggle and regain focus.

Chapter 11

Now that the diagnosis is complete, a whole new world presents itself. It is not a new and exciting world. It is a world of transition. I have to learn more about the disorder and learn how to live with it.

Gastroparesis has no cure. No one seems too sure about where it comes from. It has been linked to post gall bladder removal, chemotherapy treatment, certain medications, but nothing more specific. It has a vague link to the things mentioned but mostly the cause is unknown. Many people with gastroparesis experience nausea and vomiting. The vomiting comes often, many times a day. The stomach, still filled with old food, will reject the new food being put in, therefore causing the vomiting. Somehow I was spared this terrible experience. My body went straight to the pain portion of the symptoms list and stayed there. I was not terribly concerned with how this happened to me. I did not want to get caught up in the "why me?" I just needed to know what to do with it now.

The eating is definitely a problem. With the foods one must avoid: fat, chocolate, fiber, how is one supposed to gain weight? Then there are the amounts that one can eat. When one takes two or three bites of something non-fat every two or three hours, well, weight gain is laughable. I have now resorted to baby foods and graduate meals. Then there is the pureed food to consider. Ugh. Most foods are just not even close to appetizing when pureed. But that does not matter so much as whetting the appetite is not a concern for someone with gastroparesis. The brain closes its link to hunger. When doing something causes pain every time it is done, then the brain stops desiring that something in a classic situation of self-preservation. The brain protects the individual from the pain and discomfort.

But let's be honest, eating is a nightmare. Small portions. Nothing is appealing. I am not ever hungry. Eating because you have to, instead of because you want to, takes all the fun out of food. I also have four grown children, a husband, the girlfriend of one of our sons, and a three-year-old grandchild in the house. There is plenty of food. All kinds of food from great dinners to tasty snacks but none of it is for me. My husband and I used to have a weekly night out. Just us, without the kids. We would go to dinner, and then maybe do some shopping. We used to go, get a coffee and a bagel, and sit at the park and just people watch. It was our time. Quiet time, just for us. We do not do that anymore. Eating out is a waste of money because I don't eat. Going shopping takes so much energy out of me that it becomes a chore instead of an activity of enjoyment. Sitting at the park and watching others do what I can no longer do is just depressing. I am not who I used to be. I am at a crossroad in my life and I struggle each day with what to do next.

Oddly enough, I spend a lot of time cooking and baking. I know that sounds almost insane but it works for me for a variety of reasons. Cooking and baking allows me to have control in an area of my life where I no longer have control. I cook the things I would like to eat, but can't. I can move slowly and take breaks as I need to. I can do it sitting down. There is no rush. Also since I am not going to eat it I can put any ingredient in that I need to. I can make high-fat high-calorie foods and never have to worry. No guilt! My family has put on weight but not me. I cook for others as well. I can find pleasure in their pleasure. I can cook to help someone out who is not feeling well or overwhelmed with daily stress, or I can cook for someone just because I want to. Before this happened, I never enjoyed cooking. I knew how to cook but simply derived no pleasure from it. Back then, I would not cook things that I did not like. If I wouldn't eat it, I wouldn't cook it. Now I cook everything, whether I like it or not. It no longer matters because the cooking is for someone else's pleasure.

The difficulty of this crossroad that I find myself at is that I am not, nor ever will be, who I was before. I am an active person. My husband used to call me his "energizer wife." I enjoyed being busy. No job was too hard or too big or too dirty. Together my husband and I remodeled our whole house. I don't mean we planned it and hired someone. Nor do I mean we painted. I mean we stripped each room down to the studs. We planned and budgeted and did all the work ourselves. We did wiring, plumbing, sheet-rocking, flooring, wood work, windows, and decorating all ourselves. And we enjoyed doing it.

In my career as a nurse, again there was no job too big or too dirty. As the manager at a nursing school, there were challenges every day. There was high stress but great rewards watching students achieve their dream. In nursing, something new is always coming around. Greater resources and treatments are always on the horizon. I loved being a part of that world. Now I can no longer keep up with the pace. I do not know who the new me will be but I will continue the struggle until I can find my way into this new world. I can only hope that pain-free living and pain-free eating, even if in small portions, will come. Maybe this nightmare will end in a new and beautiful dream.

The horizon for me maybe only as far as Pennsylvania. There is a doctor there that can perform a procedure to insert a gastric pacemaker. It works like a heart pacemaker using electrical impulses to stimulate the muscles of the stomach. It may not change how I can eat but it has been reported to eliminate the pain. There is always hope.

Epilogue

I have read several stories of other people diagnosed with this disorder and they seemed to have gone through the same kind of needless suffering. I am a nurse with many friends who are also nurses. With all the support, advice, and connections within this group of people, I still had a great amount of difficulty navigating through the system. I feel horrified thinking of how people with no medical background navigate through the system. Blind trust in this system could be fatal. I have family and friends that have the same type of personality I have. As I said I am assertive. I do not just blindly follow. I ask questions, I point out inconsistencies, and I point out inadequacies. I try to point these things out using logic and a smile, but that does not always work. If I, and my family and friends had such a hard time, how bad is it for others? What about the elderly or the soft-spoken person? How about parents trying to advocate for their children? Do they too all face the same struggle?

Our current health care system is designed to make money, avoid lawsuits, and protect the staff. The patient is last on the list of priorities. It has become such a liability to provide care that the safest action is now inaction. This is an absolute outrage. Patients have become victims. Recovery from illness or injury must be more luck and happenstance than true medicine.

Our system needs to change. It has known this for many years but followed its own prescription of inaction. People need to speak out. Ask questions. Demand quality care. Hold the health care system accountable. The health care system is a monster that has broken free and is no longer under any kind of control. A change needs to occur, whether by force or by choice. Either way the current method is atrocious and it is surprising to me that anyone actually gets better after accessing this monster.